Skin Care Tips and Diet Guide

Made Handy - Beauty Edition

By

CYNTHIA LEONARD

Table Of Contents

INTRODUCTION: UNDERSTANDING YOUR SKIN

The Anatomy of Skin

The biggest organ in the human body, the skin is crucial for the body's defence against the environment, temperature control and sensory perception. It has many levels, each of which has a distinct structure and purpose. An overview of the skin's anatomy is given below:

Epidermis:

The skin's epidermis is its topmost layer.

The stratum corneum, which is the top layer, the stratum granulosum, the stratum spinosum, and the stratum basale, also known as the stratum germinativum, are some of the sublayers that make up this layer.

The majority of the epidermis is made up of keratinocytes, which create the protein keratin, which gives the skin its tensile and waterproofing qualities.

Melanin, a pigment that gives skin its colour and provides protection from UV rays, is produced by melanocytes, which are found in the stratum basale. The epidermis contains immune cells called Langerhans cells that aid in pathogen defence.

Dermis:

The layer below the epidermis is called the dermis and it contains connective tissue, blood vessels, nerves and a variety of accessory structures.

Fibres of collagen and elastin found in it provide the skin strength, suppleness and support.

The dermis contains hair follicles, sweat glands, sebaceous (*oil*) glands and nerve endings.

By contracting or expanding to store or release heat, blood vessels in the dermis control body temperature.

Hypodermis / Subcutaneous Tissue:

The skin's lowest layer, the hypodermis, is found underneath the dermis. It is made up of blood vessels, nerves and adipose (*fat*) tissue.

The hypodermis serves as an insulator, assisting in controlling body temperature while cushioning and protecting underlying components.

Auxiliary Structures:

Hair Follicles: Hair follicles may be seen extending into the subcutaneous tissue from the dermis. Sebaceous glands are connected to them and they create hair.

Sweat glands *(also known as sudoriferous glands):* These glands cause sweating, which aids in controlling body temperature and removing waste.

Sebaceous Glands: Sebaceous glands release sebum, an oily material that moisturises and protects the skin and hair from drying out.

Nails: At the base of each nail, there is a nail matrix, which is a specialised structure composed of keratin that lies under the epidermis.

Arteries and Nerves:

Blood arteries that assist feed cells and control temperature are abundantly present throughout the skin.

The feeling of touch, warmth, pressure and pain is made possible by sensory nerve endings in the skin.

The intricate structure and functions of the skin make it an essential organ for preserving general health and wellbeing. To keep the skin healthy and intact, it must be properly cared for and protected.

What's Your Skin Type?

Knowing your skin type is mandatory for choosing the right skincare products and routines since it may assist you in addressing certain issues and maintaining healthy skin.

The various prevalent varieties of skin, includes:

Ordinary Skin:

- Skin that is normal is balanced, neither overly greasy or dry.

- It is often devoid of imperfections, has a smooth texture and tiny pores.

- Normal skin usually feels loose and elastic, not tight or oily.

Greasy Skin:

- Excess sebum produced by oily skin may result in a glossy complexion and enlarged pores.

- Acne and blackheads are more common in those with oily skin.

- A good skincare regimen may reduce excessive oil production and stop pimples.

Dry Skin:

- Lacking moisture, dry skin might feel tight, flaking or scratchy.

- It could be more sensitive, prone to irritation, and prone to redness.

- Moisturisers and hydrating creams are crucial for treating dry skin.

Skin Type: Combination

A blend of several skin types on various places of the face is known as combination skin.

The cheeks may be dry or normal, but the T-zone (*forehead, nose and chin*) is often greasy.

Skincare that is tailored is required to treat both oily and dry regions.

Skin Sensitivity:

Redness, pain and irritation are common with sensitive skin.

Different skincare products and environmental variables might have a detrimental effect on it.

For sensitive skin, gentle, fragrance-free and hypoallergenic products are often advised.

Skin Prone to Acne:

Skin that is prone to acne is more likely to break out often and to produce cysts, whiteheads, blackheads and pimples.

Acne management strategies include proper washing and acne-fighting substances.

Ageing / Mature Skin:

Age-related skin changes such as fine lines, wrinkles and lack of suppleness are visible in mature skin.

Retinol and hyaluronic acid are two anti-aging substances that may assist in addressing these issues.

Dehydrated Skin:

Even though the skin isn't necessarily dry, dehydrated skin is devoid of fluids.
It could look drab and feel constricting.
Dehydration may be treated with hydrating products and plenty of water consumption.

Skin Types: Normal to Sensitive

This skin type combines minor sensitivity with normal skin. People who fall under this group could sometimes get red or irritated.

Rosacea-Predisposed Skin:

Rosacea is a skin disorder that causes facial flushing, redness and visible blood vessels.

Rosacea symptoms may be managed with the use of certain skincare products and treatments.

You may develop a customised skincare regimen that meets your requirements by knowing your skin type and any particular skin conditions you have. To maintain healthy, bright skin, it's important to choose components and products that are appropriate for your skin type.

Do speak with a dermatologist or skincare expert for advice and suggestions if you're unclear of your skin type or have particular skincare issues.

Common Skin Issues

People of various ages and socioeconomic levels often worry about skin problems. A few of the most typical skin conditions are:

Acne: Acne is a common skin ailment that develops when oil and dead skin cells block hair follicles. With it, pimples, blackheads and whiteheads are often the outcome. It may be minor or severe.

Eczema: A collection of skin illnesses known as eczema (*dermatitis*) create red, itchy and inflamed skin. Numerous things, including allergies, irritants and heredity, might cause it.

Psoriasis: Psoriasis is a long-term autoimmune disorder that results in a fast turnover of skin cells and the development of thick, scaly areas of skin. It often manifests as elevated, crimson plaques that are coated in silvery scales.

Rosacea is a long-lasting skin disorder that causes facial redness, flushing, and clearly visible blood vessels. In certain situations, it may also result in acne and eye discomfort.

Dermatitis is a broad word for skin irritation that may be brought on by allergies (*allergic dermatitis*) or contact with irritants (*contact dermatitis*). Soaps, detergents and certain plants are some common irritants.

Hives (*Urticaria*): Hives are red, itchy welts that may occur quickly and are often brought on by stress or an allergic response. They normally disappear in a few days to a few hours.

Skin infections may be caused by bacterial, viral or fungal infections. Impetigo, herpes, ringworm and cellulitis are a few typical instances.

Warts: Human papillomavirus (HPV) is the virus that causes warts, which are non-cancerous growths. They may affect many different body areas and are often infectious.

Sunburn: Overexposure to the sun's ultraviolet (UV) rays may result in sunburn, which causes red, itchy skin and raises the risk of developing skin cancer.

Skin Cancer: Skin cancer, such as melanoma, basal cell carcinoma and squamous cell carcinoma, may arise through repeated exposure to sunlight or from other causes. Treatment and early diagnosis are essential.

Dry Skin: Environmental causes, ageing or underlying medical issues may all contribute to dry skin. It may cause pain, flaking and irritation.

Allergic responses: When exposed to allergens, such as foods, medicines or environmental contaminants, some people may have skin responses like hives, rashes or itching.

Scars and keloids: Injuries or medical operations may leave behind scars. Keloids are enlarged, elevated scars that have grown outside of the initial incision site.

Skin changes brought on by ageing: As individuals become older, their skin naturally changes to include wrinkles, fine lines, sagging and age spots.

A dermatologist or other healthcare professional should be consulted for an accurate diagnosis and course of therapy for skin conditions.

Medication, lifestyle modifications and appropriate skincare practices may manage or treat a variety of skin disorders. In addition, keeping healthy skin generally and using proper sun protection may aid in the prevention of several skin issues.

The Importance of a Healthy Diet for Skin

Maintaining the health and look of your skin requires a nutritious diet. The biggest organ in your body, your skin acts as a barrier against harmful outside elements like UV radiation, pollution and infections. For the skin to operate properly, proper nourishment is necessary. In order to maintain good skin, a balanced diet is crucial for the following reasons:

Supply of Nutrients: Essential fatty acids, vitamins, minerals and other nutrients are all necessary for healthy skin. These vitamins and minerals provide a young look by repairing and regenerating skin cells and maintaining skin suppleness.

Vitamins A, C, E, and K, zinc, selenium and omega-3 fatty acids are typical skin-friendly nutrients.

Production of Collagen: Collagen is a protein that gives the skin its structural support. Collagen production depends on vitamin C, which is present in fruits and vegetables. Vitamin C-rich foods may help prevent wrinkles and drooping skin.

Proper hydration is necessary for healthy skin. By keeping the skin's moisture levels balanced, water helps avoid dryness, flakiness and the development of fine wrinkles. Your skin can stay hydrated from the inside out by drinking enough water and eating meals like fruits and vegetables that are high in water content.

Antioxidants included in certain foods, such as beta-carotene, lycopene and polyphenols, may help shield the skin from UV ray damage. Sunburns, skin cancer risk and early ageing are all consequences of exposure to UV radiation.

Green tea, tomatoes and other foods high in these antioxidants, including carrots, may provide some natural sun protection.

Controlling inflammation: Skin conditions including eczema, psoriasis and eczema may all be attributed to chronic inflammation. While a diet heavy in anti-inflammatory foods like fruits, vegetables and omega-3 fatty acids may help decrease skin inflammation, a diet high in processed foods, sweets and bad fats can actually increase inflammation.

Wound Healing: Protein intake must be sufficient for both skin restoration and wound healing. Building blocks for collagen and new skin tissue synthesis are provided by protein.

Your diet should include lean sources of protein such lean meats, poultry, fish and lentils.

Skin problems: A person's diet may have an impact on some skin problems, such as acne. Some people may experience relief from some skin disorders by avoiding particular trigger foods or allergens, even though the connection between diet and skin conditions is complicated and varies from person to person.

PART 2: How Diet Affects Your Skin

Your skin's health and look are significantly influenced by your diet. The general health, texture, and look of your skin may be affected by what you consume in both good and negative ways. Some effects of nutrition on skin are:

Hydration: Keeping your skin moisturised requires drinking enough water each day. Dehydration may cause dry, flaky skin and accentuate wrinkles and fine lines. A healthy complexion and skin suppleness are maintained with proper hydration.

Nutrient Intake: Consuming a diet that is well-balanced and rich in the necessary nutrients is key for having good skin. Several essential nutrients are:

- **Vitamins:** Vitamins including A, C, and E aid in collagen formation, skin regeneration and defence against environmental harm.

- ***Omega-3 Fatty Acids:*** These good fats, which may be found in fish, flaxseeds and walnuts, can lessen inflammation and keep the moisture in the skin.

- ***Antioxidants:*** Foods high in antioxidants, such as fruits, vegetables and green tea, fight free radicals, which may hasten the ageing process and harm skin.

- ***Zinc:*** Zinc promotes skin recovery and aids in controlling oil production.

Inflammation: Certain diets, especially those heavy in sugar, refined carbs and saturated fats, may cause the body to become inflamed. Chronic inflammation may hasten skin ageing and aggravate skin diseases like rosacea and acne.

Glycemic Index: Meals having a high glycemic index, such as processed meals and sugary foods, may cause blood sugar levels to jump. These increases may cause more oil to be produced, which may aggravate acne.

Food Sensitivities and Allergies: Some people may have skin responses, such as hives or eczema, that are brought on by certain food allergies or sensitivities. Skin health may be improved by identifying and avoiding certain trigger foods from your diet.

Production of Collagen: Collagen is a protein that maintains skin elastic and young-looking. Lean meats, salmon and soy are examples of foods high in amino acids that may help in collagen formation.

Coffee and Alcohol: Drinking too much coffee and alcohol may cause dehydration and dilated blood vessels, which can make problems like redness and puffiness worse.

Salt Intake: High salt consumption may cause water retention, which can result in puffy eyes and a bloated look.

Dietary Supplements: To promote the health of their skin, some people take dietary supplements like biotin, collagen or vitamin E. However, it's crucial to speak with a doctor before taking supplements since too much of them might have negative consequences.

Food Allergies and Acne: For some individuals, eating meals with a high glycemic index or those containing dairy might make their acne worse. The connection between nutrition and acne, however, differs from person to person.

A well-balanced diet consisting of a range of foods high in nutrients, plenty of water and moderate intake of processed and sugary foods helps support healthy and youthful skin. It's important to keep in mind that different people may have different skin sensitivities to certain foods, so observing how your skin reacts to your diet may help you make tailored decisions for improved skin health. It is advised to seek guidance from a dermatologist or other healthcare provider if you have certain skin disorders or issues.

Essential Nutrients for Skin Health

A nutritious diet that is balanced is necessary for maintaining good skin. These nutrients have a number of functions that support skin health, including healing sun-damaged skin, guarding against UV damage and maintaining young, moisturised skin. The following nutrients are crucial for healthy skin:

Vitamin C: Vitamin C is an antioxidant that aids in defending the skin from free radical damage brought on by pollutants and UV radiation. Additionally, it promotes collagen synthesis, which is necessary for skin firmness and suppleness. Vitamin C-rich foods include broccoli, bell peppers, strawberries, citrus fruits and strawberries.

Vitamin E: Another potent antioxidant, vitamin E may lessen the effects of ageing and protect the skin from oxidative damage. Avocado, spinach, nuts, seeds and seeds are excellent sources of vitamin E.

Vitamin A: Vitamin A is essential for the growth and maintenance of skin cells. It lessens the possibility of acne and helps to prevent dry skin. Dark leafy greens, sweet potatoes and carrots all contain beta-carotene, which the body may convert into vitamin A.

Vitamin D: Vitamin D promotes the health of the skin generally and may be used to treat psoriasis. Sunlight exposure, fortified meals and supplements are all ways to get it.

Omega-3 Fatty Acids: These good fats support the lipid barrier of the skin, which keeps the skin moisturised and stops moisture loss. Walnuts, flaxseeds, and fatty fish *(such as salmon and mackerel)* are excellent providers of omega-3s.

Zinc: Zinc is necessary for the repair of skin and may lessen the symptoms of acne. Additionally, it promotes the growth of fresh skin cells. Beans, whole grains and nuts are foods high in zinc.

Biotin: Also referred to as vitamin H, biotin is necessary for strong, healthy skin, hair and nails. Biotin may be found in whole grains, eggs and nuts.

Protein called Collagen: Collagen gives the skin structure. Consuming meals high in amino acids like glycine, proline and lysine may boost collagen formation even if collagen cannot be obtained directly from diet. These amino acids may be found in bone broth, poultry, fish and beans.

Staying hydrated is essential for maintaining healthy skin. Water keeps the skin's natural moisture balance in check and keeps it appearing supple and young.

Antioxidants: Beta-carotene and selenium, in addition to vitamins C and E, may aid in preventing skin damage. Beta-carotene is found in orange and yellow fruits and vegetables, while selenium is found in Brazil nuts.

Silica: A trace mineral known to improve skin hydration and suppleness is silica. Oats, brown rice and whole grains contain it.

Protein: Protein is necessary for the synthesis of collagen and elastin, two substances that preserve the firmness and suppleness of the skin.

Include lean protein sources in your diet, such as chicken, fish, tofu and lentils.

Foods to Avoid for Better Skin

While certain foods might worsen skin conditions or cause breakouts, others can encourage smooth, healthy skin.

The following meals should be avoided for healthy skin:

Sugary Foods: Consuming excessive amounts of sugar may cause inflammation and glycation, which destroys collagen and elastin and causes early ageing and acne. Limit your intake of sweets, drinks and sugary snacks.

Processed Foods: Foods that have been heavily processed often include artificial chemicals, preservatives and harmful trans fats that may aggravate acne and cause skin irritation. Instead, choose full, unadulterated meals.

Dairy Products: For some individuals, dairy triggers acne or exacerbates pre-existing skin issues. Try switching to dairy-free substitutes like almond milk or coconut yoghurt if you think dairy could be a problem.

High Glycemic Foods: Foods with a high glycemic index, such as white bread, sugary cereals and white rice, may cause blood sugar levels to surge, which may aggravate acne and other skin conditions.

Fried Meals: Fried meals often include harmful fats that may worsen skin conditions and irritation. Instead, go for culinary techniques like baking, steaming or grilling.

Fatty Meat Cuts: Regularly eating fatty meats might increase sebum production, cause inflammation and even make acne worse. Choose leaner meat cuts or think about getting your protein from plants.

Alcohol: Alcohol may cause the skin to become dehydrated and expand blood vessels, which makes it seem red and puffy. Additionally, excessive alcohol use might deny your body of certain nutrients that are necessary for good skin.

Caffeine: While modest amounts are usually okay, too much caffeine will dry out your skin. Make sure to drink lots of water in addition to any caffeine you may consume.

Spicy Meals: Spicy meals may increase skin blood flow, causing possible irritation and increased skin redness. If you see that eating spicy foods makes your skin condition worse, you may want to reduce your consumption.

Salt: Too much salt may cause water retention and puffiness, which can dull the appearance of your skin. Watch how much salt you consume, particularly if you tend to swell easily.

Foods that are Allergenic: Some individuals may be allergic or sensitive to certain foods, such nuts, shellfish or gluten, which may show up as skin problems. Consult a healthcare provider if you think a certain diet is the source of your skin issues.

Consider substituting skin-friendly items in your diet for these meals that irritate the skin. Fruits, vegetables, lean meats and whole grains are examples of foods high in antioxidants, vitamins and minerals that help enhance glowing skin.

Furthermore, keeping the health of your skin depends on consuming sufficient water to remain hydrated.

PART 3: Daily Skin Care Routine

Cleansing Your Skin

Every skincare programme should start with cleansing your skin. It helps maintain your skin clean and clear by removing dirt, oil, makeup and other pollutants from its surface. In addition to reducing the risk of skin infections, proper washing may also help other skincare products work better. *Here's how to efficiently wash your skin:*

Select the Correct Cleanser:

Identify the best cleanser for your skin type. There are cleansers designed for combination, dry, sensitive and oily skin. In case you are doubtful, you may ask a dermatologist for advice.

Cleaning Your Hands

Make sure your hands are clean before touching your face to prevent spreading dirt or germs to your skin.

Remove makeup if necessary:

If you use makeup, remove it carefully before cleaning using micellar water or a makeup remover. This guarantees that your cleanser can properly remove makeup as well as clean your skin.

Freshen Your Face:

To moisten your face, give it a splash of warm water. Use cool water instead of hot since hot water may dry out your skin by removing its natural oils.

Utilise a cleaner:

Apply a tiny quantity of the cleanser of your choice gently on your face. Apply with your fingers in an upward, circular motion. Strict rubbing or scrubbing should be avoided since it might irritate the skin.

Cleanse completely:

Pay close attention to the T-zone, which consists of the chin, forehead and nose. Be careful while around the sensitive eye region. It's important to wash your neck as well since it's often forgotten.

Rinse:

Make sure to thoroughly rinse off the cleanser from your skin with lukewarm water. A residue that is left on the skin might irritate it.

Dry Off:

Apply a clean, soft cloth to your face and gently pat it dry. Avoid touching your skin since doing so may lead to friction and possible harm.

Add toner afterwards (optional):

To balance the pH levels of the skin, some individuals prefer to use a toner after cleaning. If you decide to use a toner, use a cotton pad or your fingers to apply it.

Moisturise:

Apply a moisturiser appropriate for your skin type after cleaning and, if necessary, toning. Your skin retains and retains moisture when you moisturise.

Use sunscreen in the morning:

Apply a broad-spectrum sunscreen after cleaning your face in the morning to shield your skin from UV ray damage.

To keep good skin, you must wash your face twice daily—in the morning and just before night. You may obtain a bright and beautiful complexion by regularly washing your skin and combining it with other skincare routines like exfoliation and enough hydration. Additionally, do remember any particular skin disorders or issues you may have since these may call for specialised washing procedures or products.

Choosing the Right Cleanser

A crucial part of any skincare regimen is picking the appropriate cleanser for your face. Without irritating your skin or upsetting its natural balance, the appropriate cleanser may help remove dirt, makeup, excess oil and pollutants from your skin. Some suggestions to assist you in selecting the best cleanser for your face:

Predict Your Skin Type:

- How oily, dry, combo, sensitive or normal is your skin? The kind of cleanser that is best for you may depend on your skin type.

- A foamy or gel cleanser may be beneficial for oily skin.

- A creamy or moisturising cleanser may be preferred by dry skin.

- Use a mild, well-balanced cleanser for combination skin.

- A cleanser that is hypoallergenic, fragrance-free, or mild is necessary for sensitive skin.

Keep Harsh Ingredients Out:

Look for a cleanser devoid of harsh substances like sulphates (SLS, SLES), alcohol and artificial perfumes since these may irritate your skin and strip it of its natural oils.

pH-Equal Cleansers:

It's crucial for the health of your skin to preserve the natural acid mantle by using a pH-balanced cleanser (pH 5.5). Your skin won't get too acidic or alkaline thanks to it.

Examine Your Skincare Objectives:

Choosing a cleanser that tackles your particular skincare problems, like acne, ageing or hyperpigmentation, may be a good idea.

For instance, a cleanser containing salicylic acid may aid skin that is prone to acne, while a cleanser with antioxidants may be beneficial for skin that is becoming older.

Asthma and Sensitivities:

Read the ingredient list carefully if you have allergies or sensitivities to any particular substances. Look for products with labels that say they are hypoallergenic or safe for skin that is sensitive.

Patch test:

Conduct a patch test on a small area of skin before using a new cleanser to your full face to check for any negative reactions or allergies.

Formulation and Texture:

Take into account the cleanser's texture and composition. Cleansers with cream are hydrating, while those with foam might be more energising. Micellar water is a mild alternative for speedy makeup removal, while gel cleansers are appropriate for oily skin.

Solar Protection:

Some cleansers may include additional sunscreen components for enhanced protection, but this is not a replacement for using actual sunscreen. Use a different sunscreen cream throughout the daytime at all times.

Budget:

The cost of skincare items might vary significantly. Pick a cleanser that is within your price range and yet satisfies your skincare requirements.

Obtain a dermatologist's advice:

Consider seeing a dermatologist if you have complicated skin issues or disorders. Based on the particular requirements of your skin, they may provide tailored advice.

Do not forget that a good cleanser is just one component of your skincare regimen. For full skincare, use a suitable moisturiser and sunscreen thereafter. For the greatest effects, use your selected cleanser every day as part of your skincare regimen; consistency is also important.

Proper Cleansing Techniques

Proper washing is essential for a skincare routine, as it helps clean the skin of debris, oil, makeup and pollutants. To ensure proper cleansing, start by washing your hands thoroughly with soap and water before touching your face.

Choose a cleanser appropriate for your skin type, such as micellar water cleansers, gel, cream or foam. For sensitive skin, use a mild cleanser without scent.

Use lukewarm water instead of hot water to avoid drying up the skin and removing its natural oils. Remove makeup first using a makeup remover or washing oil to avoid blocked pores.

Gently apply the cleanser to your face, avoiding too much scrubber. Focus on key areas like the forehead, nose, chin (*T-zone*) and hairline region.

Use a gently exfoliating tool or a soft silicone face washing brush for improved cleansing. Rinse your face with lukewarm water and ensure no cleanser residue remains. After cleaning, gently wipe your face dry with a clean cloth. Apply a toner to balance pH levels and a moisturiser to seal in moisture.

Ideally, wash your face twice daily, either in the morning or before bed. Exfoliate your skin 1-2 times each week, depending on your skin type, before using additional skincare products to eliminate dead skin cells.

Avoid over-cleansing to maintain skin's natural oils and prevent dryness. Customise your skincare regimen for your unique skin type and issues.

PART 4: Exfoliation - Removing Dead Skin Cells

Benefits of Exfoliation

Exfoliation is the procedure used to remove dead skin cells from your skin's surface. It has a number of advantages for the condition and look of your skin. The following are some of the main advantages of exfoliation:

Improved Skin Texture: Exfoliation makes your skin feel softer and looks more luminous by helping to smooth out rough and uneven skin texture.

Enhanced Skin Clarity: Exfoliation may enhance skin clarity and lessen the appearance of blemishes, acne and blackheads by eliminating dead skin cells and unclogging pores.

Increased Skin Cell Turnover: Exfoliation improves the skin's natural renewal process by encouraging the formation of new, healthy skin cells. This may make your skin seem younger and more vibrant.

Reduced Fine Lines and Wrinkles: By increasing collagen synthesis and skin suppleness, regular exfoliation may help decrease the appearance of fine lines and wrinkles.

Better Product Absorption: Skin that has just been exfoliated is more responsive to skincare products, enabling serums, moisturisers and other treatments to absorb deeper and be more efficient.

Brighter Composure: Exfoliation may aid in the fading of dullness, hyperpigmentation and dark spots, resulting in a skin tone that is lighter and more even.

Ingrown Hair Prevention: Exfoliating the skin before shaving or waxing may help prevent ingrown hairs by removing any impediments to hair growth.

Reduced Oiliness: Exfoliation may reduce excessive oil production, which is particularly advantageous for those with oily or acne-prone skin.

Smoother Shaving and Makeup Application: A smoother canvas may be created by exfoliating before shaving or applying makeup, resulting in a more pleasant shave and perfect makeup application.

Relief from Stress: Exfoliating your skin may be a soothing self-care habit that promotes wellbeing and reduces stress.

It is important to remember that there are several ways to exfoliate, including chemical exfoliation (*using acids like alpha hydroxy acids or beta hydroxy acids*) and physical exfoliation (*using scrubbing particles or tools*).

Based on your skin type and specific requirements, you should decide on the technique and frequency of exfoliation. It's crucial to utilise exfoliation products and procedures correctly and adhere to a skincare regimen that is suitable for your skin type since excessive exfoliation may cause skin irritation and damage.

Types of Exfoliants

Exfoliants come in a variety of forms, and they may be divided into two major categories: **chemical** and **physical** exfoliants. Below is a description of each kind:

Physical Exfoliants: Exfoliants that utilise physical force to remove dead skin cells are known as physical exfoliants. The skin's barrier may be harmed by over-exfoliation, thus these exfoliants should only be used carefully.

Scrubs: These products are used to scrub away dead skin cells by massaging the skin with tiny, gritty particles like sugar, salt, apricot kernels or microbeads.

- **Brushes and Scrubbing Tools:** To gently scrub the skin's surface, use facial brushes, sponges or tools like a Clarisonic.

- **Washcloths:** When cleaning the skin, a gentle washcloth may be used to physically exfoliate the surface.

- **Microdermabrasion** is an expert exfoliating method that uses a machine to spray minute abrasive crystals on the skin and then hoover them away, removing dead skin cells in the process.

Chemical Exfoliants: Chemical exfoliants break or weaken the connections between dead skin cells so that they may be more easily shed from the skin. Chemical exfoliants are often favoured because they may provide outcomes that are more regulated and reliable.

- **Alpha hydroxy acids** (AHAs) are water-soluble acids that exfoliate the top layer of skin. Examples of AHAs include glycolic acid, lactic acid and citric acid. They work well to smooth out the skin's texture and minimise the visibility of fine wrinkles.

- **Beta hydroxy acids** (BHAs) are utilised in skincare products most often as salicylic acid. It works well on skin that is prone to acne since it is oil-soluble and enters pores to help clear them.

- **Enzymes:** Enzyme exfoliants breakdown and break down dead skin cells using natural enzymes like bromelain (*from pineapple*) and papain (*from papaya*).

- **Polyhydroxy Acids** (PHAs): In comparison to AHAs and BHAs, PHAs are a softer family of chemical exfoliants with bigger molecular sizes. They are suited for skin types with sensitive skin.

- **Retinoids**: By encouraging cell turnover, retinoids like retinol and prescription-strength tretinoin indirectly aid in exfoliation and skin rejuvenation.

Exfoliation Frequency

Your skin type, the exfoliant you're using, and how much your particular skin can tolerate will all influence how often you should exfoliate. The following general recommendations for exfoliation frequency:

Normal or mixture Skin: You may normally exfoliate twice or three times each week if you have normal or mixed skin. You may use either chemical exfoliants (*products containing chemicals like alpha hydroxy acids, beta hydroxy acids or enzymes*) or physical exfoliants (*scrubs with tiny particles*).

Oily Skin: Those with oily skin may often exfoliate more regularly, at least three to four times each week. Beta hydroxy acid salicylic acid is especially useful for oily skin types.

Skin that is Dry or Sensitive: You should only exfoliate your skin once or twice a week if you have dry or sensitive skin. Use moderate enzymatic exfoliants or gentle exfoliants with a lower concentration of active chemicals.

Mature Skin: Regular exfoliation, often twice weekly, is beneficial for mature skin. Exfoliation might assist in lessening the visibility of age spots and fine wrinkles.

Acne-Prone Skin: Exfoliating more often may be beneficial for acne-prone skin, but it's vital to be careful not to overdo it since this may cause discomfort. A dermatologist can provide you with more specific advice.

Body Exfoliation: You may exfoliate your body up to 2-3 times each week. To keep your body's skin smooth, use an exfoliating glove or body scrub.

Follow these guidance for safe and efficient exfoliation:

- You should always adhere to the product's directions.

- Exfoliate gently to prevent causing harm to your skin.

- After exfoliating, use sunscreen every day to Reduce the frequency of exfoliation or switch to a softer product if you feel extreme redness, irritation or peeling.

- Lastly, it's critical to monitor your skin's reaction and modify your exfoliation programme as necessary.your skin may become more sensitive to the sun.

Hydrating and Moisturizing

Hydration and moisturization are essential components in a skincare program for maintaining healthy, glowing skin.

Hydration refers to the skin's water content, which is crucial for elasticity, suppleness and overall health. Dehydration can lead to tightness, flakiness and dullness.

External factors like climate, environmental contaminants and over-cleansing can cause skin loss. To maintain moisture, focus on hydration by consuming enough water and using moisturising products like hyaluronic acid, glycerin, aloe vera and other humectants.

Moisturising involves retaining the skin's natural moisture and preventing it from escaping into the surrounding air. It helps control oil production and maintains skin balance, even for oily skin. Occlusive ingredients in moisturisers, such as oils and butters and emollients, help lock in moisture.

Your skin type should guide your moisturiser selection. For dry skin, use a thicker, richer product, while oily skin should use a lightweight, oil-free product. To effectively moisturise and hydrate, choose a mild cleanser that won't dry out your skin, use hyaluronic acid in moisturising serums and essences and apply a moisturiser suitable for your skin type.

To prevent UV damage and early ageing, finish your morning routine with a broad-spectrum sunscreen. Use a thicker moisturiser or night cream before bed to retain moisture.

Maintaining consistency is essential, using products appropriate for your skin type and following a schedule. Remember to adjust your regimen based on your skin's needs and seasonal variations.

Selecting the Right Moisturiser

For moisturised, healthy skin, choosing the best moisturiser for your skin type and requirements is crucial. You may follow these instructions to pick the best moisturiser:

Choose Your Skin Type

Dry Skin: You most likely have dry skin if it feels tight, flaking or harsh.

Oily Skin: Oily skin may be glossy and prone to breakouts and acne.

Combination Skin: Combination skin has patches of your face that are both dry and oily.

Normal skin is described as neither being too dry nor excessively greasy.

Think about any Skin Issues

Acne-Prone: To prevent clogging pores, look for oil-free or non-comedogenic moisturisers.

Sensitive Skin: Choose hypoallergenic and fragrance-free moisturisers for sensitive skin to reduce irritation.

Ageing Skin: Pick moisturisers containing retinol or peptides, two anti-aging compounds.

Sun protection: For the best sun defence, use a midday moisturiser with SPF.

Formula and Texture

Creams: Because they are heavier and provide deep hydration, they are perfect for dry or older skin.

Lotions: Lighter than creams, lotions are good for skin types with normal to mixed skin.

Gels: Because they are light and non-greasy, they are best for skin that is oily or acne-prone.

Serums: Highly concentrated serums are excellent for tackling certain issues like fine wrinkles or discoloration.

Ingredients to Watch Out For

Hyaluronic Acid: All skin types may benefit from hyaluronic acid's ability to draw in and hold moisture.

Glycerin: An efficient hydrator that is suitable for most skin types is glycerin.

Ceramides: Excellent for dry skin, help preserve the skin's barrier function.

Antioxidants (*Vitamins C and E*): Guard against environmental harm to the skin.

SPF: UV radiation protection for daylight usage.

Avoiding Dangerous Ingredients

- Sensitive skin may get irritated by fragrances and colours.

- Avoiding alcohol in excessive doses is advised since it may be drying.

- If you are worried about potentially dangerous ingredients or have sensitive skin, it may be wise to stay away from parabens and sulphates.

Perform Patch Testing

Perform a patch test on a small area of your skin to check for bad reactions before using a new moisturiser on your face.

Review Reading and Getting Recommendations

You may find an appropriate moisturiser with the aid of online evaluations and suggestions from friends or dermatologists.

Considerations for Pricing

Not necessarily are more expensive moisturisers better. Excellent hydration and skin benefits are available from several inexpensive solutions.

Consider the Seasons

In the winter, you could want a thicker moisturiser, and in the summer, a lighter one.

Be Reliable

Over time, applying the appropriate moisturiser for your skin type might provide greater benefits.

The ideal moisturiser for you will ultimately rely on the kind of skin you have, your issues and your personal tastes. Finding the ideal product may need some trial and error, but the time spent doing so will be worthwhile for maintaining healthy, moisturised skin.

PART 5: SUN PROTECTION

Understanding Sun Damage

It's essential to comprehend sun damage if you want to keep your skin healthy. Sun damage is the term used to describe the injury done to skin as a result of exposure to ultraviolet (UV) radiation from the sun.

While some sun exposure is important for the body to synthesise vitamin D, too much or exposure without protection may cause a number of skin issues and raise the risk of skin cancer.

The following is a list of solar damage:

UVA and **UVB** are two categories of dangerous UV radiation that are emitted by the sun and have an impact on skin.

UVA Rays: These cause the skin to age more quickly than it should. They may produce wrinkles, fine lines, and age spots by thoroughly penetrating the skin.

UVB rays: These are the ones that give people sunburns. They influence the epidermis and are a key factor in the development of skin cancer.

Sun damage's effects include:

Sunburn: Sunburn is a frequent sign of too much UVB exposure and is characterised by redness, discomfort and peeling.

Premature Ageing: Long-term sun exposure hastens the ageing process of the skin, causing wrinkles, fine lines and age spots.

Skin Cancer: Melanoma, squamous cell carcinoma, and basal cell carcinoma are all types of skin cancer that are significantly at risk due to sun exposure.

Hyperpigmentation: Skin dark spots or patches may result from an overproduction of melanin brought on by sun exposure.

Actinic Keratosis: Long-term sun exposure may cause a disease called actinic keratosis, which can cause rough, scaly areas on the skin and if addressed, can progress to skin cancer.

Defending against Sun damage

Sunscreen: Even on overcast days, use a broad-spectrum sunscreen with at least SPF 30.

Sun Protective Clothing: Wear long sleeved shirts, hats with broad brims and sunglasses to protect your skin and eyes from the sun.

Seek Shade: Avoid being in the sun's direct rays from 10 am to 4 pm.

Re-Apply Sunscreen: Apply sunscreen again every two hours if you're outside and more often if you're swimming or perspiring.

Avoid Tanning Beds: Tanning beds should be avoided since they release dangerous UV rays.

Regular Skin Checks: To identify any possible problems early, do self-examinations and schedule routine visits with a dermatologist.

Taking Care of Sun Damage

Topical products: Products available over-the-counter or on prescription that include retinoids, vitamin C and alpha hydroxy acids may help certain UV damage heal.

Chemical Peels: To remove layers of damaged skin, dermatologists might use chemical peels.

Laser Therapy: Several laser procedures, including laser resurfacing and intense pulsed light (IPL) therapy, may repair sun damage.

Cryotherapy: Actinic keratoses and other precancerous skin growths may be frozen off with cryotherapy.

Maintaining healthy, youthful-looking skin while lowering the risk of skin cancer requires understanding UV damage and adopting precautions. Starting to shield your skin from the damaging effects of the sun is never too late.

Sunscreen: Your Skin's Best Friend

Sunscreen is a crucial tool for maintaining healthy skin. It protects the skin from harmful UV radiation, which can cause sunburn, premature ageing and increased skin cancer risk.

Sunscreen with a high SPF helps prevent sunburn by reducing the intensity of UVB rays that cause it. Prolonged sun exposure can cause wrinkles, fine lines, age spots and loss of suppleness. Sunscreen also reduces the risk of skin cancer by obstructing UVA photons that cause photoaging.

Sunscreen also helps maintain an even skin tone by preventing hyperpigmentation and dark patches by reducing melanin production, the pigment responsible for these abnormalities. UV radiation can damage DNA in skin cells, leading to various skin problems and disorders.

Sunscreen serves as a barrier that protects the skin's integrity and health.

Sunscreen creams are available in various formulas, including hypoallergenic, non-comedogenic and designed for specific skin issues. They are easy to incorporate into your daily skincare routine and can be used under makeup. Sunscreen is essential year-round, even on gloomy or rainy days.

It is essential to use sunscreen regardless of the season, as it can harm your skin.

Lastly, Sunscreen is your skin's greatest friend, providing protection against UV radiation's damaging effects, upholding skin health and promoting a young, even complexion.

Incorporating sunscreen into your daily skincare routine is an effective step towards healthier, more vibrant skin.

Sun Protection Tips

Here are some recommendations for sun safety:

Use sunscreen: Even on overcast days, cover all exposed skin with a broad-spectrum sunscreen with an SPF (*Sun Protection Factor*) of at least 30. Reapply at least every two hours, more if you're swimming or perspiring.

Wear protective clothes, such as long-sleeved shirts, hats with a broad brim, and sunglasses that block UV rays. Even more beneficial is clothing with a UPF (*Ultraviolet Protection Factor*) rating.

Seek Shade: Try to stay in the shadow, particularly between 10 a.m. and 4 p.m., when the sun is at its strongest. Natural UV protection is provided by the shade.

Avoid Sunlamps and Tanning Beds: Sunlamps and tanning beds generate concentrated UV radiation that may harm your skin and raise your chance of developing skin cancer.

Drink lots of water to remain hydrated since exposure to the sun might cause dehydration. Skin that is dehydrated is more vulnerable to injury.

Check UV Index: Be mindful of the UV index in your region by checking it. The danger of sunburn and skin damage increases with increasing UV index. Create a plan for your outside activities.

Protect Lips: To prevent sunburn and possible skin damage, remember to use lip balm with SPF.

Kids' Sunscreen: Apply children's sunscreen to children above the age of six and keep them well-protected with clothes and caps.

Reapply Sunscreen After Swimming: Even if the sunscreen's label says it's water-resistant, reapply it after swimming or perspiring. Sunscreen may be removed by water.

Regular Skin Check: Check your skin often for any unexpected growths, moles or modifications to moles that already present. Consult a dermatologist if you detect anything odd.

Don't Just Rely on Shade: Even if you're in the shade, objects like sand, water and concrete may still reflect UV radiation onto you. So, keep applying sunscreen.

Stay Informed: Keep up with the most recent advice and rules for sun protection. Guidelines and sunscreen formulas may change over time.

Protect Your Eyes: Wear sunglasses that completely filter UVA and UVB rays to protect your eyes from sun damage and lower your chance of developing cataracts.

Do Remember that sun protection is crucial all year round, not just in the summer. Even on cloudy days, UV radiation may get through the clouds and harm the environment. Put sun protection first if you want to keep your skin looking healthy and youthful while lowering your chance of developing skin cancer.

PART 6: TARGETED SKIN CARE TIPS

Acne Management

The most prevalent times for individuals to get acne are throughout their adolescent and early adult years. Although managing and minimising acne outbreaks may be difficult and even upsetting, there are several methods and treatments that can be used.

Here is a thorough approach on managing acne:

Keep a Good Skincare Routine:

Gentle Cleaning: To remove extra oil, debris, and dead skin cells, use a gentle, non-comedogenic (*won't clog pores*) cleanser twice a day. Avoid rough rubbing since it might aggravate acne and cause skin irritation.

Moisturising: Apply a mild, oil-free, non-comedogenic moisturiser on your skin to keep it nourished. Even if you have oily skin, you should avoid over-drying it since this might increase oil production.

Products sold over-the-counter (OTC):

Topical treatments: Look for over-the-counter (OTC) medications that have chemicals like salicylic acid, benzoyl peroxide or alpha hydroxy acids (AHAs). These have the ability to cleanse pores and lessen swelling.

Spot treatments: To target particular blemishes on individual pimples, think about using sulphur or benzoyl peroxide.

Medications on prescription:

Consult a dermatologist if over-the-counter remedies are ineffective. Stronger topical medications such as topical antibiotics, retinoids or combination solutions may be prescribed by them.

In situations with moderate to severe acne, oral antibiotics may also be administered in order to minimise inflammation and manage bacteria.

Oral contraceptives (*for females*) or isotretinoin (*Accutane*) may be advised for severe instances of hormonal acne.

Managing hormonal acne:

Hormone changes are often linked to hormonal acne. Women's hormones may be regulated with the use of birth control medications.

A dermatologist could advise the anti-androgen drug spironolactone to treat hormonal acne.

Diet and way of life:

Diet: There is some research that suggests a diet rich in fruits and vegetables and low in dairy products may help reduce acne. Consuming less sugar and processed food may also be advantageous.

Controlling stress: Stress may make acne worse. Stress management techniques include yoga, meditation and regular exercise.

Prevent Triggers:

Squeezing, popping or plucking pimples may cause scars and more irritation.

Avoid spending too much time in the sun since it might harm your skin and make acne worse. Use sunscreen constantly.

Choosing Skincare Products:

To prevent blocking pores, use skincare and cosmetics that are non-comedogenic.

To avoid bacterial growth, routinely clean makeup brushes and sponges.

Treatments by Professionals:

Acne and acne scars may be effectively treated with dermatological treatments such as chemical peels, microdermabrasion, laser therapy and extractions. The finest alternatives for your skin may be determined by seeing a dermatologist.

Consistency and Patience:

Treatment for acne takes time. With your skincare regimen and any prescription drugs, be patient and persistent.

Consult a dermatologist to look into other treatments if the first one doesn't work.

It may take some trial and error to discover the best acne treatment strategy for your unique skin type and requirements. Remember what works for one person may not work for another. The most effective strategy to create a customised acne treatment plan is often to see a dermatologist.

Causes of Acne

Although the precise aetiology of acne is not entirely known, it is thought to be the consequence of a number of different elements working together. Some of the primary causes and influencing elements of acne are:

Sebum is an oily material that the sebaceous glands in the skin create in excess. Acne may result from excessive sebum production because it can block hair follicles by mixing with dead skin cells.

Clogged Hair Follicles: When sebum and dead skin cells clog hair follicles, an environment is created where bacteria, especially Propionibacterium acnes, may flourish. Inflammation and the development of pimples may result from this.

Hormonal Changes: Hormonal fluctuations may increase sebum production and cause acne. These variations can happen during puberty, menstruation, pregnancy and certain medical diseases *(such polycystic ovarian syndrome).*

Diet: Although the link between diet and acne is still up for discussion, several studies indicate that dairy products and meals with a high glycemic index may make some people's acne worse.

Genetics: There may be a hereditary predisposition to acne given that the ailment may run in families.

Bacterial infections may cause inflammation and exacerbate acne when they exist in hair follicles.

Skin Irritation: Harsh skincare products, cosmetics, friction from clothes or accessories and acne may all aggravate skin irritation.

Medication: As a side effect, several drugs, such as corticosteroids, some oral contraceptives and lithium, may cause acne.

Stress: Although it may not be the main cause of acne, stress's effects on hormone levels and the condition of the skin as a whole may make acne worse or make it more difficult to treat.

Environmental Factors: Pollution and several environmental contaminants may aggravate acne and aggravate skin inflammation.

It is important to remember that each person's acne may vary greatly in intensity and underlying reasons. While it could be a small, transient problem for some, it might be a persistent, more serious condition for others. Effective acne management and therapy often include skincare regimens, way of life adjustments and, in some circumstances, dermatologist-prescribed medicinal treatments.

Treating and Preventing Acne

Cleaning your skin is the first step in both treating and preventing acne. Wash your face twice a day with a mild cleanser, especially in the morning and just before bed. Scrubbing too vigorously might aggravate acne and cause skin irritation.

Topical Therapies:
Products that are sold without a prescription (OTC): A number of OTC creams, gels and lotions include active chemicals including salicylic acid, benzoyl peroxide or alpha hydroxy acids (AHAs). These have the ability to destroy germs, soothe irritation and unclog pores.

A dermatologist may recommend topical antibiotics, retinoids, or other drugs to treat more severe or chronic acne if OTC remedies are ineffective.

Home remedies and way of life:

- Avoid popping or squeezing pimples; doing so may result in infection, scarring and more breakouts.

- Some research contends that diets high in processed sugar and high in glycemic index meals are associated with acne.

- Think about eating a balanced diet that includes plenty of fresh fruits, vegetables, healthy grains and lean meats.

- Stress may make acne worse. Use relaxation methods like yoga, meditation or deep breathing.

Adequate Skincare:

- *Use non-comedogenic products*: Look for sunscreen, moisturisers and cosmetics that are not pore-clogging and have the non-comedogenic label.

- *Sun protection*: Exposure to the sun may exacerbate acne and leave scars. Use an SPF of 30 or more on a broad-spectrum sunscreen.

- *Hydration*: Keep your skin moisturised by drinking plenty of water. Maintaining proper hydration may benefit skin health.

Refrain from Overwashing: Although it's necessary to keep your face clean, overwashing may dry out your skin and make acne worse. Maintain a consistent cleaning schedule.

Hormone therapy: In certain circumstances, hormonal imbalances might be a factor in acne development. A medical professional could advise birth control tablets, spironolactone or other hormonal treatments.

Professional Treatments: For more severe instances of acne, dermatologists provide numerous in-office procedures including chemical peels, microdermabrasion and laser therapy.

Acne Scar Management

Depending on the nature and severity of the scars, managing acne scars requires a variety of strategies. While certain treatments may dramatically lessen the look of acne scars, it's essential to remember that sometimes they may not be completely removed. A few typical techniques for treating acne scars:

Topical Remedies

Retinoids: By encouraging collagen formation and exfoliating the skin, topical retinoids like tretinoin may help improve skin texture and lessen the visibility of scars.

Peeling agents: By removing the top layer of skin with acids, chemical peels encourage the development of new, smoother skin. With minor scars, superficial peels could be helpful.

Microdermabrasion: The top layer of skin is removed by a machine during this operation, which may make light scars look and feel better.

Dermabrasion: Dermabrasion is a more involved process than microdermabrasion that entails using a specialised tool to remove the top layers of skin.

Microneedling: Small wounds are made in the skin by microneedling, which encourages the synthesis of collagen and helps scars heal.

Laser Treatment: Scars may be made to look less noticeable by a variety of laser procedures, including fractional laser and CO2 laser resurfacing.

Fillers: Depressed scars may temporarily be raised to the level of the surrounding skin by being filled with dermal fillers.

Gel or sheets of silicone: Scars may be flattened and softened using silicone treatments if used often over time.

Injections of steroids:
Injections of corticosteroids may assist to lessen inflammation and flatten elevated or keloid scars.

Surgery: For more severe scars, surgery such as punch excision, subcision or skin transplants may sometimes be required.

Sunscreen and skin care: To stop additional harm to the skin and enhance its general health, a good skincare regimen that consists of gentle washing, moisturising and sun protection is essential.

Professional Advice: Consult a dermatologist or skincare expert to evaluate your particular scars and choose the best course of action for your particular requirements.
Consistency and Patience:

It may take many treatments and some time for scars to improve. Be patient and persistently abide by the advice of your healthcare practitioner. Do know that different people respond differently to scar treatment and not all scars can be entirely removed. As a result, controlling expectations and getting expert advice are essential components of treating acne scars. Furthermore, refraining from popping or squeezing pimples may aid in preventing the development of new scars in the first place.

Anti-Aging Strategies

Anti-aging techniques aim to enhance physical and mental health while preventing or minimising the consequences of ageing.

These techniques include a balanced diet, regular workouts, adequate sleep, stress reduction, using sunscreen, skincare, quitting smoking, maintaining hydration, taking supplements, scheduling regular medical exams, cognitive activity, social networking, hormone therapy, proper hygiene and choosing a healthy lifestyle.

A balanced diet is essential for maintaining a healthy appearance and preventing the onset of ageing. Consume fresh produce, whole grains, lean meats and healthy fats, also take antioxidants like vitamins C and E. Stay hydrated by drinking plenty of water. Regular workouts improve cardiovascular health, bone density and muscle mass, reducing the risk of falls and injuries.

Sleep is crucial for overall well-being, with 7-9 hours of sleep per night being essential for physical and mental well-being.

Stress-reduction methods like deep breathing exercises, yoga, meditation or mindfulness can help reduce ageing. Sunscreen is essential to protect skin from harmful UV rays and reduce the risk of developing skin cancer.

Skincare regimens should include washing, moisturising, and wearing sunscreen, with products containing retinoids, hyaluronic acid and antioxidants.

Limit alcohol and refrain from smoking to prevent skin damage and ageing. Consume alcohol in moderation to maintain health.

Maintain adequate water intake to keep skin and body moistened.

Regular medical exams are essential for early identification and treatment of age-related health risks. Cognitive activities, social networking, hormone therapy and good hygiene habits can help maintain overall health as you age. Every person experiences ageing differently and genetics also play a significant role in it.

PART 7: MANAGING SKIN CONDITIONS

Eczema, Psoriasis and Rosacea

It may be difficult to manage skin problems like eczema, psoriasis and rosacea, but with the right care and treatment, you can lessen symptoms and enhance the health of your skin.

To create a specialised treatment plan, close collaboration with a medical expert, such as a dermatologist, is necessary. Here are some general pointers for dealing with these ailments:

Atopic dermatitis, often known as Eczema:

Regular moisturising will keep your skin nourished. Use a hypoallergenic, fragrance-free moisturiser every day. Itching and dryness are reduced as a result.

Avoid triggers: Recognise and stay away from substances that aggravate your eczema, such as certain foods, textiles, soaps and detergents.

Use gentle soaps: Select gentle, unscented soap, and steer clear of hot showers since they might dry up your skin.

Prescription drugs: In extreme situations, your doctor may give oral anti-inflammatory drugs, topical corticosteroids or calcineurin inhibitors.

Psoriasis:

Topical therapies: Creams and ointments with corticosteroids, retinoids or coal tar may be purchased over-the-counter or obtained by prescription to treat psoriasis symptoms.

Light therapy: For some persons with psoriasis, phototherapy with UVB or PUVA may be beneficial.

Oral or injectable medications: To reduce the immune system's reaction in extreme circumstances, your doctor may give systemic drugs such methotrexate, cyclosporine or biologics.

Practise stress management strategies like since stress may cause flare-ups of psoriasis.

Rosacea:

Use moderate, fragrance-free cleansers and moisturisers for gentle skincare. Avoid using abrasive skincare products and harsh scrubbing.

Sun protection: Use broad-brimmed hats and sunscreen with an SPF of 30 or higher to shield your skin from the sun. Sunlight exposure may make rosacea worse.

Prescription drugs: To lessen redness and inflammation, doctors may recommend oral antibiotics, azelaic acid or metronidazole as topical therapies.

Avoid triggers: Recognise and stay away from things like spicy meals, alcohol, hot drinks and high temperatures that may cause rosacea flare-ups.

Common Sense Advice for All Skin Conditions

* Drink enough water to keep your body and skin properly hydrated.

* Choose hypoallergenic, fragrance-free products for skincare and washing to avoid irritation.

* Maintain a healthy lifestyle by getting adequate sleep, engaging in regular exercise and eating a balanced diet high in fruits and vegetables.

* Work closely with a dermatologist who can keep an eye on your health and modify your treatment strategy as necessary.

Tips for Soothing Irritated Skin

Determine the reason: Make an effort to determine the reason for the irritation before using any therapies. Is it brought on by a skin disease (*such psoriasis or eczema*), an allergic response, a wound or too much sun exposure?

You can choose the best course of therapy by being aware of the reason.

Keep It Clean: Gently wash the inflamed area with warm water and a moderate, fragrance-free cleanser. Avoid using hot water or abrasive soaps since they might aggravate the skin even more.

Avoid Scratching: While it may be tempting to scratch itchy skin, doing so may aggravate the itch and perhaps cause an infection. Keep your nails short to reduce harm from scratching and try to fight the impulse.

Apply a Cold Compress: Applying a cold compress might help lessen irritation and redness. Apply a clean cloth-wrapped cold pack or some ice to the affected region for 15 to 20 minutes. A direct application of ice to the skin should be avoided as it might result in frostbite.

Use a mild, fragrance-free, hypoallergenic moisturiser to keep the skin moisturised. Look for products with ceramides, hyaluronic acid or glycerin as components. To keep moisture in your skin after washing, moisturise right away.

Avoid Irritants: Pay attention to ingredients in skincare products that might cause irritation, such as scents, alcohol and certain preservatives. Choose items with the labels "hypoallergenic" and "non-comedogenic."

Use Muesli Baths: Muesli baths may calm sensitive skin and assist to reduce itching. Oats should be ground into a fine powder and then added to a warm bath. For 15 to 20 minutes, soak.

Creams available over-the-counter (OTC): Creams containing hydrocortisone help ease inflammation and irritation. Stick to the directions on the container and refrain from using them for a lengthy amount of time or on your face without first visiting a healthcare provider.

Stay Hydrated: To keep hydrated from the inside out, drink lots of water. Skin that is well-hydrated is less irritable.

Wear Loose, Breathable Clothes: To reduce friction and irritation, pick loose-fitting, breathable materials like cotton if the irritated region is covered by clothes.

Sun Protection: Apply a broad-spectrum sunscreen with at least SPF 30 before going outdoors if the irritation is caused by a sunburn. This will shield your skin against additional UV deterioration. Wear protective clothes as well, such as long-sleeved shirts and caps with broad brims.

Consult a Dermatologist: For a correct diagnosis and treatment plan, seek the advice of a dermatologist or other healthcare expert if the irritation lasts, becomes worse or is accompanied by other alarming symptoms (*such as an infection*).

Working with a Dermatologist

Maintaining healthy skin, identifying and treating skin disorders and addressing different aesthetic issues may all be accomplished with the help of a dermatologist. Here's how to communicate with a dermatologist successfully, whether you have a particular skin issue or are interested in skincare for general wellbeing:

How to Choose a Dermatologist:

- Find a board-certified dermatologist with a solid reputation by doing some research.

- Location, accessibility and area of expertise (*medical, cosmetic, paediatric, etc.*) should all be taken into account.

Schedule a Consultation:

- If available, utilise the dermatologist's online scheduling tool or call the clinic.

- Describe your visit's purpose and any particular worries you may have.

Getting ready for the appointment:

- Make a note of your current skincare regimen, prescription drugs and any skin issues or treatments you've had in the past.

- Bring any pertinent test results or medical documents, if any.

Consultation:

- Discuss in depth your skincare objectives and worries throughout the consultation.

- Be open and truthful about your lifestyle, skincare routine and any symptoms you may be experiencing.

Examining the skin:

- To evaluate your problem, the dermatologist will probably do a comprehensive skin examination.

- To diagnose and assess your skin, they could use specialised equipment or methods.

Treatment Strategy:

Your dermatologist will create a customised treatment plan based on the evaluation.
This plan may include skincare advice, dietary suggestions, lifestyle modifications or treatments *(such as biopsies, laser therapy and chemical peels)*.

Pose queries:

- Do not be afraid to inquire about your disease, available treatments, and any adverse effects.

- If there is anything you don't understand, ask for an explanation.

Observe Directions:

- Follow your dermatologist's advice and the recommended course of therapy.

- Apply skincare products as instructed and take prescription drugs as indicated.

Track Progress:

- Observe any changes in your health and how your skin reacts to therapy.

- Inform your dermatologist right once of any issues or negative effects.

Attend Follow-Up Consultations:

- To evaluate your progress and make any required modifications to your treatment plan, follow-up meetings are crucial.

- Even if your skin seems to have gotten better, continue the suggested follow-up programme.

Just wait:

- Be patient and reasonable in your expectations since treating many skin diseases takes time.

- A dermatologist should always be consulted before using over-the-counter medications and self-diagnosing.

Keep Up Regular Check-Ups:

- It is advised to see your dermatologist for regular checkups even after your skin issue has been resolved.

- These consultations may assist with current difficulties as well as potential problems.

Open communication:

- Inform your dermatologist right once if your skin changes or if any new problems appear.

- The key to keeping good skin is clear communication.

- The healthiest skin is achievable when you work with a dermatologist to obtain and maintain it.

- You may attain the greatest outcomes and reduce skin-related issues by adhering to their advice and being active in your skincare programme.

PART 8: DIET FOR HEALTHY SKIN

Nutrients for Glowing Skin

A balanced diet, a healthy lifestyle and good skincare all play a part in achieving and preserving bright skin. The health and shine of the skin are significantly influenced by nutrients.

Here are some key vitamins and minerals for radiant skin:

Vitamin C: Vitamin C is an antioxidant that aids in defending the skin against free radical damage brought on by pollution and sun exposure. Additionally, it encourages the synthesis of collagen, which is necessary for skin firmness and suppleness.
Strawberries, bell peppers and citrus fruits are all excellent sources of vitamin C.

Vitamin E: Another antioxidant that helps preserve skin health and fight free radicals is vitamin E. It also helps to hydrate the skin. Foods including almonds, sunflower seeds and spinach contain vitamin E.

Vitamin A: Vitamin A is necessary for the development and repair of skin cells. It may assist in lessening the visibility of wrinkles and blemishes. Vitamin A is abundant in foods including sweet potatoes, carrots and leafy greens.

Omega-3 Fatty Acids: By maintaining the skin's lipid barrier, omega-3 fatty acids keep the skin moisturised and guard against dryness and irritation. Walnuts, flaxseeds and fatty seafood like salmon are great sources.

Collagen: Collagen is a protein that gives the skin its structural support. While you cannot eat collagen, you may eat foods high in the amino acids glycine, proline and lysine, which serve as the collagen's building blocks. Fish, poultry and bone broth are all excellent sources.

Zinc: Zinc is essential for healthy skin because it promotes the growth of new skin cells, the creation of collagen and the healing of wounds. Zinc may be found in foods including whole grains, nuts and lean meats.

Selenium: Selenium is an antioxidant that improves skin suppleness and aids in UV damage prevention. Seafood, Brazil nuts and sunflower seeds are excellent sources of selenium.

Biotin, sometimes referred to as vitamin H, is important for keeping strong, healthy skin, hair and nails. Whole grains, nuts and eggs are foods high in biotin.

Water: Drink enough water to maintain healthy skin. Water keeps your skin moisturised and plump and aids in toxin removal.

Antioxidants: In addition to vitamins C and E, antioxidants including coenzyme Q10, green tea extract, and resveratrol—a substance found in grapes and red wine—can shield the skin against oxidative stress and early ageing.

Protein: Enough protein must be consumed for skin cells to repair and regenerate. Include tofu, beans, lean meats, chicken, fish and seafood in your diet.

Probiotics: Skin health might benefit from a balanced gut microbiota. Yoghurt, kefir and sauerkraut are examples of foods high in probiotics that may help intestinal health.

A balanced diet that includes a range of fruits, vegetables, whole grains and lean proteins is essential for general wellbeing, even though these nutrients are crucial for skin health. Maintaining healthy skin care routines will help to achieve beautiful skin.

Vitamins, Minerals and Antioxidants

A healthy diet must include vitamins, minerals, and antioxidants since they all play a part in preserving the body's general health and wellbeing. An overview of each category is given below:

Vitamins:

Vitamins are organic substances that the body needs in little amounts to sustain a number of physiological processes.

They are divided into two groups:- Water-soluble vitamins (*such as the B-complex vitamins and vitamin C*) and fat-soluble vitamins (*such as vitamins A, D, E and K*).

Each vitamin has a distinct purpose, such as stimulating development, enhancing immunity, serving as antioxidants or aiding in different metabolic processes.

Food sources: A broad range of foods, such as fruits, vegetables, whole grains, dairy products and lean meats, contain vitamins.

Minerals:

❖ The body requires different levels of minerals, which are inorganic nutrients, for a variety of processes, including bone health, fluid balance and neuron function.

❖ Calcium, magnesium, phosphorus, sodium, potassium and chloride are important minerals.

❖ Iron, zinc, copper, selenium and iodine are examples of trace minerals, which are required in tiny amounts.

❖ Enzymes, hormones and other biological activities need minerals to work properly.

❖ Numerous foods, such as dairy products, nuts, seeds, leafy greens and lean meats, contain minerals.

Antioxidants:

Antioxidants are substances that aid in defending the body against oxidative stress, which may harm cells and have a role in a number of health problems, including ageing and chronic illnesses.

They function by scavenging dangerous chemicals known as free radicals, which are generated during typical metabolic activities and exposure to environmental elements like radiation and pollution.

Vitamins C and E, beta-carotene (*a precursor to vitamin A*), selenium and different phytochemicals included in fruits, vegetables and other plant-based diets are examples of common antioxidants.

Chronic illnesses including cancer, heart disease, and neurological disorders have a lower likelihood of development in those who consume antioxidants.

Food sources: Colourful fruits and vegetables, nuts, seeds, whole grains and certain kinds of tea are all rich sources of antioxidants.

For general health, maintain a balanced and diverse diet that contains a broad variety of vitamins, minerals and antioxidants. This may assist to avoid nutritional deficiencies and lower the chance of developing chronic illnesses.

Consult a medical expert or qualified dietitian for individualised advice on how to satisfy your nutritional requirements if you have particular dietary issues or medical problems.

Omega-3 Fatty Acids

A class of polyunsaturated fats known as omega-3 fatty acids are crucial for maintaining good health in people. Because they feature a double bond three carbon atoms away from the methyl end of the fatty acid chain, they are known as "omega-3" fatty acids.

These fatty acids have been related to multiple health advantages and are essential for many physiological functions.

Omega-3 fatty acids come in three primary categories:

The plant-based omega-3 fatty acid alpha-linolenic acid (ALA) may be found in flaxseeds, chia seeds, walnuts and hemp seeds. Because the human body cannot synthesise it and must get it from food sources, it is regarded as an essential fatty acid.

Eicosapentaenoic acid (EPA): Salmon, mackerel, sardines and trout are some examples of cold-water fatty fish that are high in EPA. It has a reputation for being anti-inflammatory and is often linked to cardiovascular health.

Docosahexaenoic acid (DHA) is a fatty acid that is also present in fatty fish, especially in high concentrations in salmon and tuna. It is a significant anatomical element of the brain and is essential for both eye health and cognitive function.

Several factors make omega-3 fatty acids crucial:

Heart Health: Studies have shown that omega-3 fatty acids, especially EPA and DHA, decrease blood pressure, cut triglycerides, and improve cholesterol profiles, all of which lessen the risk of heart disease. On blood arteries, they also have anti-inflammatory properties.

DHA is a crucial part of the membranes that line the brain cells and it's crucial for the growth and operation of the brain. Omega-3 fatty acids may boost cognitive function and have positive effects on diseases like Alzheimer's and depression.

Eye Health: DHA, which is essential for keeping excellent eyesight and avoiding eye illnesses, is present in high amounts in the retina of the eye.

Inflammation: Ailments including arthritis and inflammatory bowel illnesses may benefit from the anti-inflammatory characteristics of omega-3s, which may help decrease inflammation in the body.

Mood and Mental Health: According to some study, mood disorders including sadness and anxiety may be positively impacted by omega-3 fatty acids.

Joint Health: In situations like rheumatoid arthritis, omega-3 fatty acids may help lessen joint discomfort and stiffness.

You may increase the amount of omega-3 fatty acids in your diet by including fatty fish in your meals, eating ALA-rich foods like flaxseeds and walnuts or by taking omega-3 supplements, if your doctor advises them.

PART 9: FOODS FOR RADIANT SKIN

Skin-Friendly Fruits and Vegetables

A balanced diet full of fruits and vegetables may help you have beautiful, healthy skin. These foods are bursting with antioxidants, vitamins, minerals and other elements that support healthy skin.

Here are some foods to add in your diet that are good for your skin:

Berries: Antioxidants included in berries like blueberries, strawberries and raspberries help shield the skin from damage brought on by free radicals. Additionally, they are abundant in vitamin C, which promotes the creation of collagen.

Citrus fruits, such as oranges, grapefruits, and lemons, are rich in vitamin C, which encourages the creation of collagen and aids in skin restoration.

Avocado: Avocado is a fantastic source of vitamin E and good fats. These nutrients may lessen the appearance of wrinkles while assisting in keeping the skin moisturised.

Leafy greens like spinach and kale are abundant in vitamins A and C, which are vital for healthy skin. Additionally, they contain lutein and zeaxanthin, which shield the skin from UV deterioration.

Carrots: Beta-carotene, which the body converts to vitamin A, is abundant in carrots. Vitamin A is essential for mending tissues and keeping healthy skin.

Tomatoes: Lycopene, an antioxidant that helps shield the skin from UV rays and lowers the risk of sunburn, is abundant in tomatoes.

Sweet Potatoes: Sweet potatoes are a great source of vitamin A and beta-carotene, both of which help to maintain good skin and may even give your complexion a healthy shine.

Papaya: Papaya includes enzymes like papain that may aid in skin exfoliation and encourage a smoother complexion. Vitamins A and C are also abundant in it.

Cucumber: Cucumbers contain a lot of water, which keeps the skin moisturised. They also contain silica, which promotes the formation of collagen.

Bell peppers: Bell peppers, particularly the red and yellow types, are high in beta-carotene and vitamin C, both of which are good for the health of the skin.

Broccoli: Sulforaphane, which has been demonstrated to have anti-aging and skin-protective qualities, is abundant in broccoli and is also a good source of vitamins C, K, and A.

Pomegranate: Pomegranates are full of antioxidants and polyphenols that may protect the skin from sun damage and assist to enhance skin texture.

Watermelon: Due to its high water content and the presence of vitamins A and C, which promote good skin, watermelon is moisturising.

Kiwi: Kiwi is a fantastic source of vitamins C and E, which support collagen synthesis and healthy skin.

Almonds: Almonds are rich in vitamin E and good fats that help keep skin hydrated and shield it from UV ray damage.

To achieve and maintain glowing skin, keep in mind that a balanced diet rich in a range of fruits and vegetables is essential.

Lean Proteins for Skin Health

Lean proteins are essential for skin health, as they contribute to collagen production, repair and maintenance. Collagen, found in chicken, turkey, fish and lean cuts of cattle, helps keep skin tight and elastic, reducing the appearance of fine lines and wrinkles.

Protein is also essential for the body's ability to mend wounds and restore damaged tissue.

Omega-3 fatty acids, found in certain lean protein sources like salmon, mackerel and sardines, have anti-inflammatory and antioxidant properties, reducing inflammation and protecting the skin from oxidative damage.

Lean proteins also help stabilise blood sugar levels, limiting insulin spikes and reducing the risk of skin conditions like acne and breakouts.

Prolonged inflammation is linked to skin diseases like psoriasis, eczema and acne, also lean proteins can reduce inflammation, promoting cleaner and healthier skin.

Proper hydration is crucial for maintaining skin moisture and avoiding dryness and flakiness. A balanced diet rich in vitamins, minerals and antioxidants is essential for achieving optimum skin health.

Water: The Ultimate Skin Hydrator

Water is in fact often regarded as the best hydrator for the skin. Since it keeps your skin smooth, supple, and operating correctly, hydration is essential for keeping healthy skin. This is the reason why water is necessary for hydrating skin:

Moisture Retention: Skin is made up of cells, and for these cells to operate at their best, water is necessary. Skin cells may retain their form and structure by drinking enough water, which helps keep them from becoming dry and flaky.

Elasticity and Plumpness: Proper hydration helps the skin to be elastic and plump. Skin that is well-hydrated looks younger and fuller and is less prone to sagging and wrinkles.

Barrier Function: Water is crucial for preserving the integrity of the protective barrier that skin acts as. A well-hydrated skin barrier does a better job of keeping moisture in and hazardous things out.

Healing and Repair: Hydrated skin is better at self-repairing. When it has an appropriate moisture supply, it may heal from small wounds like cuts or scratches faster and with less scarring.

Even Skin Tone: Adequate hydration may aid in balancing out skin tone by lessening the appearance of redness and blotchiness. Additionally, it might lessen how noticeable dark stains and imperfections are.

Prevention of Dryness and Irritation: Dry, itchy and irritated skin are more common in people with dehydrated skin. These problems may be avoided by consuming enough amounts of water and utilising hydrated skincare products.

Skin problems: Dryness and dehydration may aggravate a number of skin problems, including eczema and psoriasis. The signs of these disorders may be controlled by keeping the skin well-hydrated. Although drinking water is unquestionably necessary for hydrating the skin, it's crucial to remember that keeping hydrated requires both external and internal factors:

External hydration: By using moisturisers and other hydrating skincare products, you may assist the skin's barrier to retain moisture.

Internal hydration: It's essential to consume enough water to keep your body -- including your skin -- well hydrated. To maintain skin health, try to drink enough water each day.

Water is the best hydrator for the skin since it's essential for preserving the condition, hydration and general look of the skin.

PART 10: DIET DO'S AND DON'TS

Foods to Include in Your Diet

The following meals may help you have better-looking skin:

Fruits and vegetables are abundant in vitamins, minerals, and antioxidants, which help shield your skin from the harm that free radicals may do. Choose colourful varieties like carrots, berries, oranges, spinach and kale.

Fatty Fish: Omega-3 fatty acids are abundant in fatty fish, including sardines, mackerel and salmon. These beneficial fats support the skin's lipid barrier, preserving its moisture and lowering inflammation.

Nuts and seeds are wonderful sources of vitamins, minerals, and healthy fats. Some examples are almonds, walnuts, flaxseeds, and chia seeds. They may aid in reducing inflammation and promoting healthy skin.

Whole Grains: Complex carbohydrates, which are found in whole grains like brown rice, quinoa and oats, help control blood sugar levels. Maintaining steady blood sugar is crucial since it might help with skin issues.

Green Tea: Green tea is full of catechins, which are anti-inflammatory and antioxidants that help prevent skin damage. Additionally, it could help prevent skin cancer.

Avocado: The skin is nourished and hydrated by avocado's nutritious lipids, vitamins (*particularly vitamin E*) and antioxidants.

Tomatoes: Lycopene, an antioxidant that may help shield your skin from UV rays and support a healthy complexion, is abundant in tomatoes.

Sweet potatoes: The body transforms beta-carotene, which is abundant in sweet potatoes, into vitamin A. This vitamin supports the health of the skin and keeps it supple.

Protein: The amino acids needed for the formation of collagen, which gives the skin its firmness and suppleness, are found in lean forms of protein such chicken, turkey, tofu and legumes.

Water: It's important to stay hydrated for healthy skin. Water maintains your skin moisturised and bright while also aiding in the removal of toxins from the body.

Fruits and berries: Fruits rich in antioxidants, such as blueberries, strawberries and blackberries, help fight free radicals and support youthful-looking skin.

Dark Chocolate: Dark chocolate with a high cocoa content (70 *percent or more*) has antioxidants and flavonols that, when consumed in moderation, may enhance skin hydration and shield it from UV ray damage.

Balanced diet is important and foods rich in sugar, processed foods and excessive alcohol intake must be avoided or limited since they might exacerbate skin problems.

Foods to Avoid for Clear Skin

In order to attain clean skin, some foods that are often linked to skin problems should be taken in moderation or avoided. The following foods should either be limited or avoided:

Sugar: Consuming too much sugar may raise insulin levels and cause inflammation, which can aggravate acne and other skin conditions. Consuming sugary foods and beverages in moderation is recommended, including soda, candy and pastries.

Dairy: Milk in particular has been related to acne in certain people who consume dairy products. It is believed that dairy products' growth factors and hormones are to blame for this. You can think about cutting down on dairy if you think it's harming your skin.

High Glycemic Foods: Foods with a high glycemic index (GI) may raise blood sugar levels suddenly, which may result in acne. White bread, spaghetti, sugary cereals and potatoes are a few examples. Instead, choose complex carbs and healthy grains.

Fried and Greasy meals may cause oily skin and blocked pores, as can diets heavy in harmful fats and fried foods. Your skin may look better if you consume less fried meals, quick foods and processed snacks.

Saturated and Trans fats: These fats may aggravate skin disorders like acne by promoting inflammation. Reduce your consumption of foods containing hydrogenated oils, processed meats and red meat.

Salty foods: Consuming too much salt may cause water retention and puffiness, which will make your skin seem less clear and youthful. Processed meals and snacks rich in salt should only be taken occasionally.

Alcohol: Drinking too much alcohol may dry the skin, making it seem dull and perhaps aggravating existing skin disorders. Moderately consume alcohol and drink a lot of water to keep hydrated.

Caffeine: While modest amounts are usually OK, too much caffeine may dry out the skin. Make sure you drink enough water in addition to the recommended amount of caffeine.

Spicy meals: People with sensitive skin may experience redness and irritation from spicy meals since they may widen blood vessels and cause inflammation.

Artificial Preservatives and Additives: Processed foods often include artificial preservatives and additives, which in some individuals might cause allergic responses or skin sensitivities. When possible, choose fresh, whole foods.

The link between nutrition and skin health is complicated and may differ from person to person, despite the fact that some foods may have an effect on some people's skin.

The Role of Sugar and Dairy

Dairy and sugar both have an influence on skin, albeit each individual will experience these effects differently. Their functions in skincare are broken out as follows:

Sugar:

Acne: High sugar intake, particularly from processed meals, sugary beverages and sweets, may cause blood sugar levels to rise. As a result, insulin and insulin-like growth factor 1 (IGF-1) may be released, both of which may aid in the emergence of acne.

Foods with a high glycemic index might be especially harmful. Chronic inflammation is connected to a number of skin problems, including redness, puffiness and the breakdown of collagen and elastin, which may accelerate the ageing process. Sugar can trigger inflammation in the body.

Glycation: An excessive consumption of sugar may result in glycation, a process in which sugar molecules bind to proteins like collagen and elastin and make them rigid and less functioning. This may cause the skin to droop and wrinkle.

Dairy:

Acne: Dairy consumption might exacerbate acne outbreaks in those who are sensitive to the substance. It's hypothesised that hormones in milk, such as insulin-like growth factor 1 (*IGF-1*) and androgens, may contribute to increased oil production and pore blockage. However the precise processes are not entirely known.

Due to lactose intolerance or a sensitivity to dairy proteins, dairy products may potentially exacerbate inflammation in certain individuals. **Rosacea** and **Eczema** are two skin disorders that inflammation may make worse.

Hormones: Commercial dairy products often include hormones that may disrupt your own hormonal balance, such as synthetic bovine growth hormone (*rBGH*) and naturally occurring hormones. Skin conditions like acne may be brought on by hormonal abnormalities.

Not everyone will react the same way to dairy and sugar. Genetics, general dietary habits and lifestyle choices all have a big impact on skin health and some individuals may be more susceptible to these variables than others.

If you believe that dairy and/or sugar are having an impact on your skin, you may want to attempt cutting them out of your diet and seeing how your skin reacts.

PART 11: LIFESTYLE FACTORS

Stress Management

Stress may have a big influence on the health and look of your skin, thus skin care and stress management are closely related. Your body produces stress chemicals like cortisol when you're under stress, which may cause a number of skin conditions. On the other hand, by promoting a feeling of self-care and relaxation, taking care of your skin may also aid in lowering stress.

To incorporate stress reduction into your skincare routine, create a peaceful ritual with mindful skincare routines, using a mild cleanser that doesn't remove your skin's natural oils and using a moisturiser appropriate for your skin type to properly hydrate your skin.

Use sunscreen daily, even indoors, to prevent sun damage and aggravate stress-related skin issues. A well-balanced diet rich in antioxidants,

vitamins and minerals can promote good skin
and improve your body's ability to handle stress.

Regular exercise can lower stress by boosting
the production of endorphins, which are
biologically based mood enhancers.
Exercise-induced sweating can also aid in
pore-clearing, creating better skin.

Ensure adequate sleep to prevent stress levels
from rising, which can cause dark circles under
the eyes and acne.

Incorporate **stress-reduction activities** like
yoga, deep breathing, meditation or mindfulness
into your daily routine to reduce cortisol levels
and improve skin condition. Limit your intake of
coffee and alcohol, as they can dry out your skin
and worsen stress. Seek specialist help if you
have eczema or acne and are experiencing
persistent stress.

Stay hydrated by drinking enough water
throughout the day, reduce skin irritations by
choosing skin-friendly products and incorporate

self-care practices into your daily routine, such as taking relaxing baths, using calming face masks or having a massage.

Impact of Stress on Skin

Stress can have severe long-term and short-term effects on the skin, causing various health issues. Stress can cause acne, eczema, psoriasis, premature ageing, dehydration, dryness, allergic skin responses, hindering the body's normal healing processes and causing hair loss.

The body produces more cortisol, a stress hormone, during stress, which can cause the skin to produce extra oil, which can block pores and cause acne outbreaks. Eczema and psoriasis can also worsen due to increased inflammation, irritation and pain.

Long-term stress can accelerate the skin's ageing process, leading to wrinkles, fine lines and drooping skin. Dehydration and dryness can result from the skin's inability to act as a barrier, leading to dehydrated, dry skin. Stress-related rashes, such as stress-induced dermatitis, can also result from stress. Stress can disrupt blood flow to the skin, resulting in a dull complexion and increased risk of scarring and infection.

Hair loss, including disorders like telogen effluvium, can also occur due to stress.

Note that each individual has a different association between stress and skin health and stress-reduction methods like mindfulness practices, relaxation exercises and adequate sleep can help mitigate the negative effects of stress on the skin.

Stress-Reduction Techniques

You might try the following excellent stress-reduction methods:

Deep breathing might assist your nervous system become more at ease. Try the 4-7-8 breathing technique: inhale for four counts, hold for seven, and then let out eight.

Progressive Muscle Relaxation: Contract and then release each muscle in your body, working your way up from your toes to your head. Physical stress may be relieved in this way.

Meditation for mindfulness: Mindfulness entails paying attention to the situation at hand without passing judgement. By promoting increased self-awareness, meditation may help you manage stress.

Yoga: Yoga blends physical postures with breathing techniques, meditation and stress reduction.

Exercise: Endorphins, which are endogenous mood enhancers, are released during physical exercise. Over time, regular exercise may also help you sleep better and feel less stressed.

Healthy Eating: Eating a balanced diet might help you feel happier and have more energy. Reduce your intake of sweets and caffeine, which may increase tension.

Sleep: Make sure you get plenty of good sleep. Create a relaxing sleeping environment, establish a nightly ritual, and refrain from engaging in stimulating activities just before bed.

Time management: Prioritise and organise your duties to avoid feeling overloaded. Divide complicated jobs into more manageable chunks.

Social Support: Talking to friends and family may help you feel connected and supported emotionally, which helps lower stress.

Limit Screen Time: Spending too much time on the internet, particularly social media, may cause tension and anxiety. Think about limiting screen time and engaging in digital detoxes.

Journaling: Writing down your thoughts and emotions in a journal may help you digest them and gain perspective on difficult circumstances.

Laughter: Watch a hilarious movie, hang out with people who make you laugh or take part in enjoyable activities.

Relaxation Techniques: Examine relaxation techniques including aromatherapy, visualisation and relaxing music.

Set limits: Develop the ability to say no when it's required and set limits to safeguard your time and energy.

Mindful breathing: Take brief pauses throughout the day to engage in mindful breathing exercises. Spend some time concentrating on your breathing to centre yourself.

Hobbies and Interests: Take part in the pastimes or pursuits you love. This might provide satisfaction and serve as a diversion from pressures.

Professional Assistance: If your stress is excessive or ongoing, you may want to go to a therapist or counsellor. They can provide solutions and assistance that are suited to your needs.

Time in Nature: Spending time in nature may help you relax, whether you're taking a stroll in the park or a trek in the forest.

Practice Gratitude: Reflect often on the things you have to be thankful for. This may help you divert your attention from stress and encourage a positive outlook.

Apps for relaxation and biofeedback: Using these tools, you may learn to regulate physiological processes like heart rate and muscular tension, which can help you relax.

Different methods are effective for various individuals, so you must experiment to determine your own best. The greatest substantial advantages for reducing stress may often be obtained by combining several treatments.

Sleep and Skin Health

Sleep plays a crucial role in enhancing skin health, not just through skincare programs or products. Sleep promotes skin repair and regeneration, enhancing collagen production and preventing damage from environmental elements like UV radiation and pollutants. Proper circulation of blood to the skin leads to a more even complexion, ensuring skin cells have the necessary nutrients and oxygen.

Sleep deprivation can result in dark circles and puffiness, as blood vessels beneath the eyes enlarge and appear dilated.

Chronic sleep deprivation can also lead to accelerated skin ageing, causing collagen and elastin fibres to break down, resulting in wrinkles and fine lines.

Lack of sleep can also lead to skin disorders like acne, as stress can cause hormonal changes that may aggravate acne. Sleep is essential for preserving skin moisture levels, as dry and lifeless skin may result from insufficient sleep.

Skin barrier function is essential for protecting against irritants and halting moisture loss. To improve skin health, spend **7-9** hours each night getting a good night's sleep, establish a regular sleep routine, create a soothing sleep ritual and use blackout curtains, a quiet room, and a comfortable mattress. Avoid using screens before bed to disrupt the sleep-wake cycle.

The Importance of Beauty Sleep and Sleep-Enhancing Tips

The significance of beauty sleep:

Skin Care: Sleep is essential for the renewal of skin cells. The body makes collagen when you are sleeping deeply, which keeps your skin supple and young. Sleep deprivation may cause early ageing, wrinkles and a lifeless complexion.

Physical Well-Being: Physical well-being depends on getting enough sleep. It enables the body to heal and regenerate, which is essential for a number of physiological processes including immune system operation, hormone balance and muscle recovery.

Sleep is necessary for sustaining healthy mental health, according to research. Mood changes, elevated stress, anxiety and melancholy may result from sleep deprivation. A good night's sleep aids in emotional control and improves memory and problem-solving skills in the brain.

Weight management: Sleep is important for controlling hunger and metabolism. Lack of sleep increases the risk of weight gain and makes it more difficult to control weight.

Energy and Productivity: A restful night's sleep leaves you feeling reenergized and ready to take on the day, making you more productive. Lack of sleep might affect one's ability to concentrate, focus, and work efficiently.

Tips for Increasing Sleep:

Create a Schedule: Attempt to have a consistent bedtime and wake-up time each day, including weekends. This aids in regulating the biological clock in your body.

Establish a peaceful bedtime routine by partaking in activities that are calming before going to sleep, such as reading, having a warm bath or practising deep breathing.

Reduce Screen Time: The blue light that computers, tablets and phones generate may disrupt your sleep. At least an hour before night, stay away from devices.

Make your bedroom dark, quiet and at a pleasant temperature to promote restful sleep. A quality mattress and set of pillows may also make a big impact.

Watch Your Diet: Stay away from coffee, alcohol, and big meals just before night. These chemicals may interfere with sleep cycles.

Get Regular Exercise: Regular exercise might help you sleep better. Try to avoid doing vigorous activity just before bed, however.

Manage Stress: To quiet your thoughts before bed, try stress-reduction exercises like progressive muscle relaxation, yoga or meditation.

Limiting naps is important since they might disturb nocturnal sleep, even though quick power naps can be rejuvenating. If you must snooze, limit it to no more than 30 minutes.

Limit liquid intake before bed: Limit liquid intake in the hours before bed to reduce overnight awakenings for toilet breaks.

Seek practitioner Assistance: If you often struggle to fall asleep, speak with a medical practitioner or a sleep specialist. Specialised therapy may be needed for sleep problems including insomnia or sleep apnea.

Beauty sleep is essential to overall health and is not merely a notion for aesthetic purposes. You may enjoy a variety of physical, mental and emotional advantages by prioritising and improving the quality of your sleep, which adds to a better and happier existence.

Exercise for a Healthy Complexion and How it Benefits the Skin

Your skin's health in general and your complexion in particular may be greatly influenced by exercise. The following workouts are good for your skin and help to promote healthier skin:

Workouts for the heart:

Benefits: Cardio workouts like jogging, cycling, and swimming improve blood circulation, which helps the skin cells get more oxygen and nutrients. This aids in the elimination of trash and pollutants.

Improved blood flow provides your skin a healthy shine, encourages the synthesis of collagen and aids in cell regeneration, decreasing the indications of ageing.

Yoga:

Benefits: Yoga lowers stress, which may lead to skin conditions like eczema and acne. It also improves posture and flexibility.

Reduced stress may result in fewer breakouts and a more even complexion, which is beneficial for the skin. Wrinkles brought on by drooping skin may be avoided by improving posture.

Exercise for Strength:

Benefits: Resistance workouts, such bodyweight exercises or weightlifting, improve muscular growth and speed up metabolism.

A higher metabolism may aid in maintaining a healthy weight and lower the chance of developing skin disorders like cellulite. Your skin may seem firmer if your muscles are in better shape.

Face-moving exercises:

Benefits: Specific facial workouts may improve circulation in the face and tone facial muscles.

How it improves the skin: Increasing blood flow to the face with facial workouts may result in a more youthful look, less puffiness, and improved skin suppleness.

Breathing deeply:

Benefits: Deep breathing techniques assist enhance lung function, lower stress levels and soothe the mind.

How it helps your skin: Less stress may result in less cortisol being produced, which can help you have clearer skin and fewer breakouts.

Posture Correction:

Benefits: Good posture may aid in preventing skin conditions brought on by friction or pressure, such as acne mechanical (*a skin condition brought on by pressure*).

Having proper posture may help your skin by lowering your risk of breakouts and skin irritation on your chest and back.

Exercise and hydration:

Benefits: Preventing dehydration and keeping your skin moisturised by drinking water before, during, and after exercise.

How it improves the skin: Proper hydration supports the preservation of skin elasticity and a radiant, healthy complexion.

Regular exercise may enhance your complexion by boosting collagen formation, lowering stress levels and enhancing blood circulation.

For the greatest results in obtaining and preserving healthy and glowing skin, combine exercise with a balanced diet, enough hydration and a skincare programme.

PART 12: NATURAL AND DIY SKIN CARE

Homemade Skin Care Recipes

Making your own skincare products at home may be a cheap and enjoyable method to take care of your skin. Everyone's skin is unique, therefore it's vital to remember that what works for one person may not work for another.

Always do a tiny skin patch test before using any new ingredients or recipes to be sure you won't experience any negative side effects.

The following DIY skincare recipes may be used for a variety of things:

Cleansers:

Honey Cleanser: Combine honey and coconut oil in an equal ratio. After massaging your face, rinse with warm water.

Muesli Cleanser: Make a paste of oats and water. Rinse after giving your face a gentle massage.

Exfoliators:

Sugar Scrub: To make a scrub, combine sugar (*white or brown*) with olive oil or honey. After giving your skin a gentle massage, rinse.

Coffee scrub: Combine yoghurt or coconut oil with coffee grinds. After applying in a circular motion, rinse.

Masks:

Apply a mashed-up ripe avocado to your face for an avocado mask. Rinse after 15-20 minutes of application.

Yoghurt and Honey Mask: As a mask, combine yoghurt and honey in an equal amount. After 15 to 20 minutes, rinse.

Turmeric Mask: Yoghurt, turmeric and honey are combined to make a turmeric mask. Rinse after 10-15 minutes (*caution: turmeric may temporarily discolour your skin*).

Apply a mashed-up banana on your face for a mask. Rinse after 15-20 minutes of application.

Toner:

Apple cider vinegar toner: Combine water and apple cider vinegar in equal amounts. After cleaning, use a cotton ball to apply the toner. If it's too powerful for your skin, dilute it.

Moisturisers:

Coconut Oil Moisturiser: As a moisturiser, use coconut oil sparingly. Particularly beneficial for dry skin.

Aloe Vera Gel: Use pure aloe vera gel to moisturise your face. It moisturises and calms.

Serums:

Aloe vera gel or water may be added to vitamin C powder to make a serum. To increase collagen formation and brighten your skin, dab a little on your face.

Sunscreen:

Zinc Oxide Sunscreen: To make a natural sunscreen, combine zinc oxide powder and a moisturiser.

The Lip scrub:

Brown Sugar Lip Scrub: To make a lip scrub, combine brown sugar with honey or coconut oil. Use it to gently exfoliate your lips.

Eye Lotion:

Apply a tiny quantity of cucumber and aloe vera gel blended together to the area around your eyes to minimise puffiness.

Masks for Battling Acne:

Clay mask: To make a paste, use bentonite or kaolin clay with water or apple cider vinegar. Rinse after applying on blemishes and letting it sit till it dries.

Moisturising Face Mist:

Rosewater and Glycerin Mist: In a spray bottle, combine rosewater and glycerin in equal parts. Use it as a cooling spray to moisturise your skin all day long.

Age-Reducing Measures:

Brew green tea and let it cool to use as a toner. For a cooling and anti-aging effect, use it as a toner or freeze it in ice cube trays to apply on your face.

Apply vitamin E oil directly to areas with fine lines or wrinkles by puncturing the vitamin E capsule.

Body Scrub:

Lemon Sugar Body Scrub: To make a revitalising body scrub, combine sugar, lemon juice and olive oil.

Soak Feet:

Epsom Salt Foot Soak: To ease pain and soften skin, dissolve Epsom salt in warm water and soak your feet in it.

Hair Mask:

Honey and Coconut Oil Hair Mask: Combine the two ingredients and apply the mask to your hair. 30 minutes should pass before shampooing.

Hand Lotion:

Melt shea butter and combine it with a few drops of your preferred essential oil to make shea butter hand cream. Use it as a nourishing hand cream after allowing it to set.

Spray of Lavender for Pillows:

Lavender Pillow Spray: In a spray bottle, combine water and a few drops of lavender essential oil. Before going to bed, spritz your pillow with a relaxing sleep aid.

Cream for Stretch Marks:

Melt cocoa butter and include a few drops of vitamin E oil to create a cream. To areas that are prone to stretch marks, use this mixture.

Always use caution while using essential oils since they may be strong and irritating to certain people. To avoid deterioration and retain the efficacy of these manufactured items, careful storage is also crucial.

Last but not least, remember that even while DIY skincare recipes might be helpful for many individuals, they are not a substitute for expert skincare guidance.

Popular Essential Oils for Skin Care

While essential oils may be a useful addition to your beauty regimen, it's crucial to utilise them correctly and properly. Popular essential oils for skincare include the following:

Lavender Oil: The relaxing and soothing effects of lavender oil are well recognised. Minor burns, skin rashes and skin redness may all be treated with it.

Tea tree oil: Tea tree oil is excellent against acne and other skin problems because of its potent antibacterial and anti-inflammatory effects.

Frankincense Oil: Frankincense oil may help make scars, fine lines and wrinkles seem less noticeable. Additionally, it possesses anti-inflammatory qualities.

Rosehip Oil: Due to its high vitamin and antioxidant content, this oil is excellent for moisturising the skin and minimising the effects of ageing.

Chamomile Oil: The calming properties of chamomile oil are good for sensitive or irritated skin. Eczema and dermatitis are two disorders it may treat.

Jojoba Oil: Jojoba oil is a natural oil that closely mirrors the oils in our skin. For moisturising without blocking pores, it's a fantastic option.

Oil of Geranium: Geranium oil helps balance oily skin and provide a radiant appearance.

Carrot Seed Oil: Rich in vitamins and antioxidants, carrot seed oil may help tone and revitalise the skin.

Helichrysum Oil: This oil may be used to lessen the visibility of scars and blemishes and is well renowned for its ability to heal wounds.

Ylang-Ylang Oil: Ylang-Ylang oil is popular for its pleasant scent and its ability to balance the skin's oil production.

Rose oil: Rose oil is well recognised for its capacity to moisturise and calm the skin. It also has anti-aging effects.

Neroli Oil: Made from orange flowers, neroli oil is regarded for enhancing skin suppleness and minimising the visibility of scars.

Before applying essential oils to your skin, don't forget to dilute them with a carrier oil *(such jojoba, coconut or almond oil)*, since undiluted essential oils may be extremely powerful and may irritate the skin.

Using a new essential oil, it's advisable to do a patch test on a tiny patch of skin to be sure you won't have any negative side effects. Also certain essential oils may increase your skin's sensitivity to sunlight, so use caution and apply sunscreen as required while using them throughout the day.

CONCLUSION

Creating Your Personalized Skin Care Plan

To achieve healthy, bright skin, it is essential to develop a customised skincare routine. This involves determining your skin type, which can be normal, mixed, sensitive, oily or dry.

Identify your specific skin issues, such as sensitivity, pigmentation, redness, fine wrinkles, acne or fine lines and choose the appropriate products.

To clean your skin, use a mild cleanser twice daily, in the morning and before going to sleep. Exfoliate 1-3 times a week, using physical or chemical exfoliants like scrubs or AHAs.

Moisturise your skin with a suitable moisturiser, even for oily skin. Use broad-spectrum sunscreen with at least SPF 30 protection to prevent early ageing and skin damage.

Incorporate targeted therapies, such as serums or treatments designed for individual skin conditions, such as Vitamin C serums for brightening and hyaluronic acid for hydration.

Use eye creams specifically designed for eye problems, such as puffiness, dark circles or fine wrinkles around the eyes.

At night, focus on restoring and reviving your skin with a bedtime moisturiser and consider retinol or other treatments for your skin conditions.

Consult a dermatologist for specialised advice or prescribed products for conditions like acne, rosacea or hyperpigmentation.

Consistency is crucial, so follow your skincare regimen religiously and allow products time to absorb. Patch test new products on a small area of skin to avoid allergic reactions or allergies.

A good diet and lifestyle decisions are essential for maintaining healthy skin. Adjust your skincare regimen as needed due to seasonal and ageing changes. Seek professional advice for personalised evaluation and advice if you're unclear about your skin type, issues or the best products to use.

Setting Realistic Goals and Tracking Your Progress

For the results you want and to keep your skin healthy and beautiful, it's crucial to set reasonable objectives and monitor your skincare progress.

Decide What Skincare Issues You Have:

Determine your unique skincare issues first. Do you want to deal with acne, lessen fine lines and wrinkles, level out your skin ton or enhance the general health of your skin? You may make specific objectives by being aware of your main problems.

Do Your Own Research and Education:

Learn about the components and products that may help with your issues and your skin type. If necessary, get advice from a dermatologist or skincare expert to receive tailored suggestions.

Define Specific, Realistic Goals:

Make sure your objectives for your skincare routine are SMART—specific, measurable, realistic, relevant and time-bound. An example of a SMART goal might be to *"reduce acne breakouts by* **50%** *in three months by using a consistent skincare routine."*

Select the Proper Ingredients and Products:

Choose skincare components and products that support your objectives. For instance, seek for creams with components like vitamin C or niacinamide if you want to lessen hyperpigmentation.

Establish a Skincare Regime:

Make sure to incorporate cleaning, exfoliating, moisturising and UV protection in your daily and weekly skincare regimen. The secret to attaining your skincare objectives is consistency.

Beginning a Skincare Journal:

Keep a notebook to record your skincare regimen, including the items you use, the steps you follow and any alterations you make. Keep track of any advancements or setbacks in the health of your skin.

Photograph the Before-and-After:

Take pictures of your development before and after. You may evaluate the changes in your skin over time using this visual record.

Be Patience:

Be aware that benefits from skincare may not be immediate. Being patient and sticking to your programme can help you observe benefits that might often take weeks or even months to manifest.

Change Your Routine as Necessary:

Keep an eye on how your skin reacts to various products and adjust as required. Consider trying another product if one irritates you or doesn't get the results you want.

Consult a Professional:

Consult a dermatologist if you're not making the improvements you anticipated or if you have serious skin problems. If necessary, they may provide advice, advocate sophisticated procedures or prescribe certain therapies.

Uphold a Healthful Lifestyle:

Keep in mind that skin care involves more than simply products. Healthy skin is a result of a balanced diet, appropriate hydration, frequent exercise and restful sleep. Don't forget to include these elements in your regimen.

Honour Accomplishments:

Any skincare accomplishments should be celebrated. You may increase your motivation and maintain your commitment to your skincare objectives by recognising your progress.

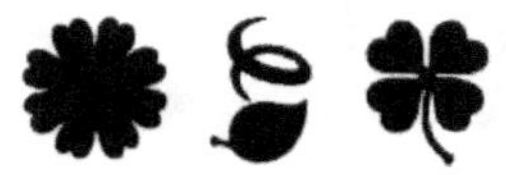